The Inspired Keto Diet Cooking Guide

Fit and Healthy Irresistible Recipes To Boost Your Brain and Fast your Metabolism

Otis Fisher

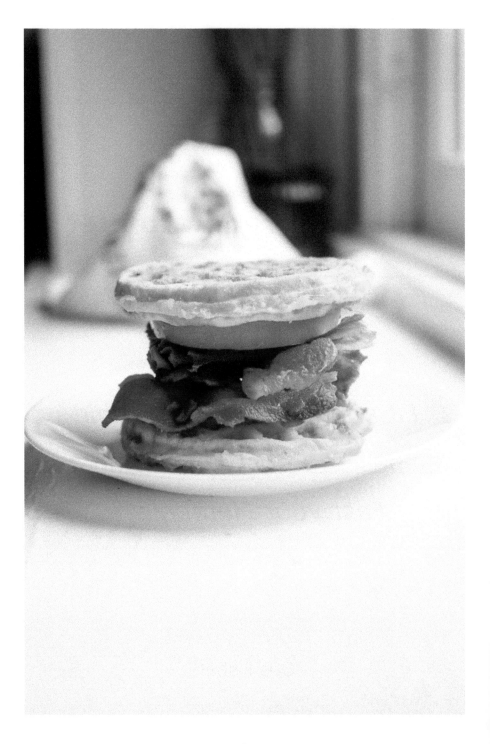

3

acknowledge that the author is not engaging in the rendering of legal, financial, medical or professional advice. The content within this book has been derived from various sources. Please consult a licensed professional before attempting any techniques outlined in this book.

By reading this document, the reader agrees that under no circumstances is the author responsible for any losses, direct or indirect, which are incurred as a result of the use of information contained within this document, including, but not limited to, — errors, omissions, or inaccuracies.

Table of contents

Tomato Pizza with Strawberries

Preparation time: 9 minutes

Cooking Time: 40 Minutes

Servings: 4

Ingredients:

- 3 cups shredded mozzarella
- 2 tbsp. cream cheese, softened
- 3/4 cup almond flour
- 2 tbsp. almond meal 1 celery stalk, chopped
- 1 tomato, chopped
- 1 tbsp. olive oil
- 2 tbsp. balsamic vinegar
- 1 cup strawberries, halved
- 1 tbsp. chopped mint leaves

Directions:

1. Preheat oven to 390 F. Line a pizza pan with parchment paper. Microwave 2 cups of mozzarella cheese and cream cheese for 1 minute.
2. Remove and mix in almond flour and almond meal. Spread the mixture on the pizza pan and bake for 10 minutes. Spread remaining mozzarella cheese on the crust. In a bowl, toss celery, tomato, olive oil, and balsamic vinegar. Spoon the mixture onto

the mozzarella cheese and arrange the strawberries on top.

3. Top with mint leaves. Bake for 15 minutes. Serve sliced.

Nutrition:

Cal 306

Net Carbs 4g

Fats 11g

Protein 28g

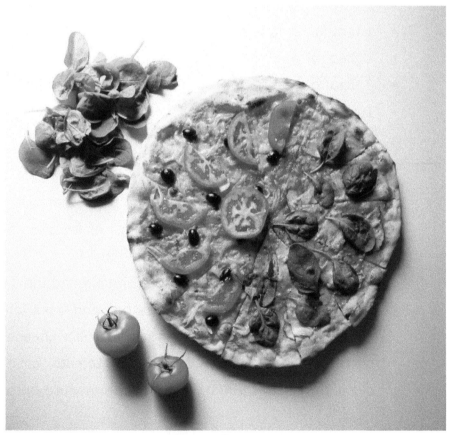

Broccoli "Rice" with Walnuts

Preparation time: 15 minutes

Cooking Time: 25 Minutes

Servings: 4

Ingredients:

- 2 heads large broccoli, riced
- 2 tbsp. butter
- 1 garlic clove, minced
- 1/4 cup toasted walnuts, chopped
- 4 tbsp. sesame seeds, toasted
- 1/2 cup vegetable broth
- 2 tbsp. chopped cilantro
- Salt and black pepper to taste

Directions:

1. Melt butter in a pot and stir in garlic. Cooking until fragrant, for 1 minute and add in broccoli and vegetable broth. Allow steaming for 2 minutes.
2. Season with salt and pepper and Cooking for 3-5 minutes. Pour in walnuts, sesame seeds, and cilantro. Fluff the rice and serve warm.

Nutrition:

Cal 239

Net Carbs 3g

Fat 15g

Protein 9g

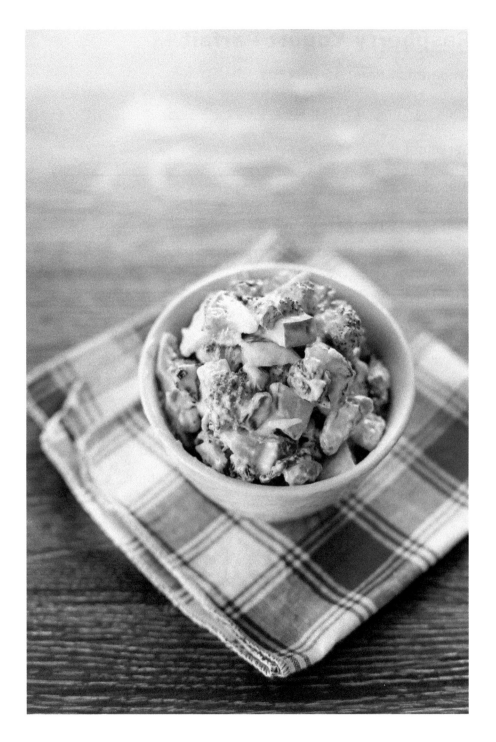

Raspberry Yogurt Parfait

Preparation time: 15 minutes

Cooking Time: 15 Minutes

Servings: 2

Ingredients:

- 1 cup Greek yogurt
- 1 cup fresh raspberries
- 1/2 lemon, zested
- 3 mint sprigs, chopped
- 2 tbsp. chia seeds
- 2 drops liquid stevia

Directions:

1. In a small bowl, set the Greek yogurt with stevia. In medium serving glasses, layer half of the Greek yogurt, raspberries, lemon zest, mint, chia seeds, and drizzle with maple syrup. Repeat with another layer.
2. Serve cold.

Nutrition:

Cal 183

Fat 10g

Net Carbs 8.9g

Protein 7.8g

Quick Beef Carpaccio

Preparation time: 9 minutes

Cooking Time: 10 Minutes

Servings: 4

Ingredients:

- 1/2 lemon, juiced
- 2 tbsp. olive oil
- 1/4 cup grated Parmesan chees
- 1/4 lb. rare roast beef, sliced
- 1 1/2 cups baby arugula
- Salt and black pepper to taste

Directions

1. Merge the olive oil, lemon juice, salt, and pepper in a bowl until well combined. Spread the beef on a large serving plate, top with arugula and drizzle the olive oil mixture on top.
2. Sprinkle with grated Parmesan and serve.

Nutrition:

Cal 112

Net Carbs 4g

Fat 5g

Protein 9g

Tomato Bruschetta with Basil

Preparation time: 9 minutes

Cooking Time: 1 hour 20 Minutes

Servings: 4

Ingredients:

- 5 tbsp. olive oil
- 3 ripe tomatoes, chopped
- 6 fresh basil leaves
- 1 garlic clove, halved
- 4 slices zero carb bread, halved
- Salt to taste

Directions:

1. In a bowl, mix tomatoes and basil until combined. Drizzle with 2 tbsp. olive oil and salt; do not stir. Set aside. Garnish bread slices with the remaining olive oil, arrange on a baking sheet, and place under the broiler. Cooking for 2 minutes per side or until lightly browned.
2. Transfer to a plate and rub garlic on both sides. Cover with tomato topping. Drizzle a little more of olive oil on top to serve.

Nutrition:

Cal 209

Net Carbs 2.7g;

Fat 17g

Protein 8g

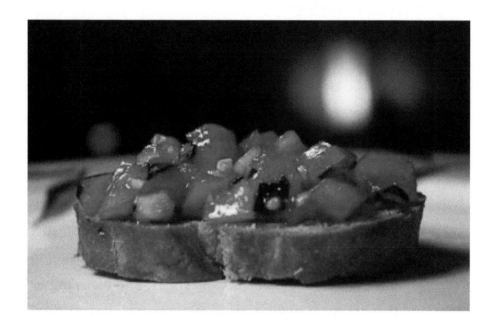

Golden Saffron Cauli Rice

Preparation time: 15 minutes

Cooking Time: 35 Minutes

Servings: 4

Ingredients:

- A pinch of saffron soaked in 1/4-cup almond milk
- 1 tbsp. butter
- 2 tbsp. olive oil
- 6 garlic cloves, sliced 1 yellow onion, thinly sliced
- 2 cups cauli rice
- 1/4 cup vegetable broth
- 2 tbsp. chopped parsley
- Salt and black pepper to taste

Directions:

1. Warm olive oil in a saucepan over medium heat and fry garlic until golden brown but not burned; set aside. Add butter to the saucepan and sauté onion for 3 minutes. Stir in cauli rice. Remove the saffron from the milk and pour the milk and vegetable stock into the saucepan. Mix, cover, and Cooking for 5 minutes.
2. Season with salt, black pepper, and parsley. Fluff the rice and dish into serving plates. Garnish with fried garlic and serve.

Nutrition:

Cal 89

Net Carbs 5.9g

Fat 6g

Protein 2g

Simple Strawberry Mousse

Preparation time: 15 minutes

Cooking Time: 28 Minutes

Servings: 4

Ingredients:

- 12 strawberries, hulled
- 1/2 cup softened cream cheese
- 1 cup heavy whipping cream
- 2 tbsp. swerve sugar

Directions:

1. Reserve some strawberries for topping. In a food processor, blend the remaining strawberries and swerve sugar until smooth. Add cream cheese and process until smooth.
2. Pour in the heavy cream and blend smoothly too. Divide the mousse into 4 medium glasses and refrigerate for 1 hour. Top with strawberries and serve.

Nutrition:

Cal 199

Net Carbs 4.7g

Fat 20g

Protein 3g

Kale and Mushroom Pierogis

Preparation time: 10 minutes

Cooking Time: 45 Minutes

Servings: 4

Ingredients:

- 7 tbsp. butter
- 2 garlic cloves, minced
- 1 small red onion, chopped
- 3 oz. belle mushrooms, sliced
- 2 oz. fresh kale
- Salt and black pepper to taste
- 1/2 cup cream cheese
- 2 cups Parmesan, grated
- 1 tbsp. flax seed powder
- 1/2 cup almond flour
- 4 tbsp. coconut flour
- 1 tsp. baking powder

Directions:

1. Melt 2 tbsp. of butter in a skillet and sauté garlic, red onion, mushrooms, and kale for 5 minutes. Season with salt and pepper and reduce the heat to low. Stir in cream cheese and 1/2 cup of Parmesan cheese; simmer for 1 minute. Set aside to cool. In a bowl, mix flax seed powder with 3 tbsp. water and

allow sitting for 5 minutes. In another bowl, combine almond and coconut flours, salt, and baking powder. Put a pan over low heat and melt the remaining Parmesan cheese and butter.

2. Turn the heat off. Pour the flax egg in the cream mixture, continue stirring, while adding the flour mixture until a firm dough forms. Mold the dough into balls, place on a chopping board, and use a rolling pin to flatten each into 1/2 inch thin round piece. Spread a generous amount of stuffing on one-half of each dough, fold over the filling, and seal the dough with fingers. Brush with foil and bake for 20 minutes at 380 F.

Nutrition:

Cal 540

Net Carbs 6g

Fat 47g

Protein 18g

Prosciutto-Wrapped Chicken with Asparagus

Preparation time: 10 minutes

Cooking Time: 45 Minutes

Servings: 4

Ingredients:

- 4 chicken breasts
- 8 prosciutto slices
- 4 tbsp. olive oil 1 lb. asparagus spears
- 2 tbsp. fresh lemon juice
- Romano cheese for topping

Directions

1. Preheat oven to 400 F. Flavor chicken with salt and pepper and wrap 2 prosciutto slices around each chicken breast. Arrange on a lined with parchment paper baking sheet, drizzle with oil, and bake for 25-30 minutes.
2. Preheat grill. Brush asparagus spears with olive oil and grill them for 8-10 minutes, frequently turning until slightly charred. Detach to a plate and drizzle with lemon juice. Grate over Romano cheese and serve with wrapped chicken.

Nutrition:

Cal 468

Net Carbs 2g

Fat 38g

Protein 26g

Cheesy Muffins with Ajillo Mushrooms

Preparation time: 10 minutes

Cooking Time: 45 Minutes

Servings: 6

Ingredients:

- 1 1/2 cups heavy cream
- 5 ounces mascarpone cheese
- 3 eggs, beaten 1 tbsp. butter, softened
- 2 cups mushrooms, chopped
- 2 garlic cloves, minced

Directions:

1. Preheat oven to 320 F. Insert 6 ramekins into a large pan. Add in boiling water up to 1-inch depth. In a pan over medium heat, warm heavy cream. Set heat to low and stir in mascarpone cheese; Cooking until melted. Place beaten eggs in a bowl and place in 3 tbsp. of the hot cream mixture; mix well. Place the mixture back to the pan with hot cream/cheese mixture. Sprinkle with pepper and salt. Ladle the mixture into the ramekins.
2. Bake for 40 minutes. Melt butter in a pan and add garlic and mushrooms; sauté for 5-6 minutes. Top the muffins with the mushrooms.

Nutrition:

Cal 263

Net Carbs: 6g

Fat: 22g

Protein: 10g

Cauliflower and Seitan Cheese Bake

Preparation time: 10 minutes

Cooking Time: 40 Minutes

Servings: 4

Ingredients:

- 2 cups broccoli florets
- 1 cup cauliflower florets
- 2 cups crumbled seitan
- 2 oz. butter
- 1 leek, coarsely chopped
- 1 onion, coarsely chopped
- 1 cup coconut cream
- 2 tbsp. mustard powder
- 5 oz. grated Parmesan
- 4 tbsp. fresh rosemary

Directions:

1. Preheat oven to 450 F. Put half of butter in a pot over medium heat to melt. Add leek, onion, broccoli, and cauliflower and Cooking until the vegetables have softened, about 6 minutes. Transfer them to a baking dish.
2. Melt the remaining butter in a skillet over medium heat, and Cooking seitan until browned. Mix coconut cream and mustard powder in a bowl. Pour mixture

over the veggies. Scatter seitan and Parmesan on top and sprinkle with rosemary. Bake for 15 minutes.

Nutrition:

Cal 479

Net Carbs 9.8g

Fat 39g

Protein 16g

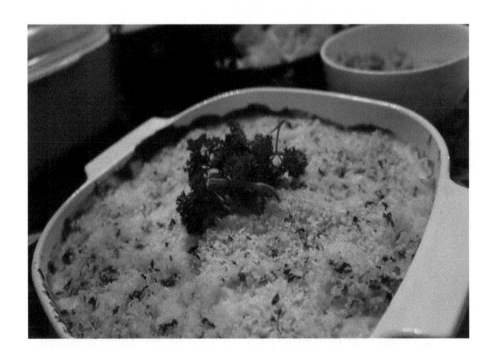

Easy Lamb Kebabs

Preparation time: 10 minutes

Cooking Time: 25 Minutes

Servings: 4

Ingredients:

- 1 pound ground lamb
- 1/4 tsp. cinnamon
- 1 egg
- 1 grated onion
- Salt and black pepper to taste
- 2 tbsp. mint, chopped

Directions

1. Set all ingredients in a bowl; mix to combine. Divide the meat into 4 pieces. Shape all of the meat portions around previously-soaked skewers. Preheat grill to medium heat. Grill the kebabs for 5 minutes per side.
2. Serve warm.

Nutrition:

Cal 467

Net Carbs 3.2g;

Fat 37g

Protein 27g

Basic Keto Pizza Dough

Preparation time: 10 minutes

Cooking Time: 15 Minutes

Servings: 8

Ingredients:

- 3 cups almond flour
- 3 tbsp. ghee
- 1/4 tsp. salt
- 3 large eggs

Directions:

1. Preheat oven to 350 F. In a bowl, mix almond flour, ghee, salt, and eggs until a dough forms. Mold the dough into a ball and place between 2 wide pieces of parchment paper on a flat surface. Use a pin roll it out into a circle of a quarter-inch thickness.
2. Slide the dough into the pizza pan and remove the parchment papers. Bake for 20 minutes. Decorate with your favorite topping and bake further.

Nutrition:

Cal 151

Net Carbs: 2g

Fat: 11g

Protein: 7g

Cheesy Brussels Sprouts Salad

Preparation time: 10 minutes

Cooking Time: 35 Minutes

Servings: 6

Ingredients:

- 2 lb. Brussels sprouts, halved
- 3 tbsp. olive oil
- Salt and black pepper to taste
- 2 1/2 tbsp. balsamic vinegar
- 1/4 red cabbage, shredded
- 1 tbsp. Dijon mustard
- 1 cup Parmesan, grated
- 2 tbsp. pumpkin seeds, toasted

Directions:

1. Warmth oven to 400 F. Line a baking sheet with foil. Garnish Brussels sprouts with olive oil, salt, pepper, and balsamic vinegar in a bowl and spread on the baking sheet.
2. Bake for 20-25 minutes. Transfer to a salad bowl and mix in red cabbage, mustard, and half of the cheese. Sprinkle with the remaining cheese and pumpkin seeds and serve.

Nutrition:

Cal 210

Net Carbs 6g

Fat 18g

Protein 4g

Tomato Bites with Vegan Cheese Topping

Preparation time: 10 minutes

Cooking Time: 15 Minutes

Servings: 4

Ingredients:

- 2 spring onions, chopped
- 5 tomatoes, sliced
- 1/4 cup olive oil
- 1 tbsp. seasoning mix For vegan cheese
- 1/2 cup pepitas seeds
- 1 tbsp. nutritional yeast
- Salt and black pepper, to taste
- 1 tsp. garlic puree

Directions

1. Drizzle tomatoes with olive oil. Preheat oven to 400 F. In a food processor, add all vegan cheese ingredients and pulse until the desired consistency is attained. Combine vegan cheese and seasoning mix. Toss in the tomato slices to coat.
2. Set tomato slices on a baking pan and bake for 10 minutes. Top with spring onions and serve.

Nutrition:

Cal 161

Net Carbs: 7g

Fat: 14g

Protein: 5g

Salami Cauliflower Pizza

Preparation time: 10 minutes

Cooking Time: 45 Minutes

Servings: 4

Ingredients:

- 2 cups grated mozzarella
- 4 cups cauliflower rice
- 1 tbsp. dried thyme
- 1/4 cup tomato sauce
- 4 oz. salami slices

Directions:

1. Preheat oven to 390 F. Microwave cauliflower rice mixed with 1 tbsp. of water for 1 minute. Remove and mix in 1 cup of the mozzarella cheese and thyme.
2. Pour the mixture into a greased baking dish, spread out and bake for 5 minutes. Remove the dish and spread the tomato sauce on top. Scatter remaining mozzarella cheese on the sauce and then arrange salami slices on top. Bake for 15 minutes.

Nutrition:

Cal 276

Net Carbs 2g

Fats 15g

Protein 20g

Baked Cheese and Cauliflower

Preparation time: 10 minutes

Cooking Time: 30 Minutes

Servings: 4

Ingredients:

- 1 head cauliflower, cut into florets
- 1/4 cup butter, cubed
- 2 tbsp. melted butter
- 1 white onion, chopped
- 1/4 almond milk
- 1/2 cup almond flour
- 1 1/2 cups grated Colby cheese

Directions:

1. Preheat oven to 350 F. Microwave the cauli florets for 4-5 minutes. Melt the butter cubes in a saucepan and sauté onion for 3 minutes. Add in cauliflower, season with salt and pepper, and mix in almond milk. Simmer for 3 minutes.
2. Mix the remaining melted butter with almond flour. Stir into the cauliflower as well as half of the cheese. Sprinkle the top with the remaining cheese and bake for 10 minutes. Plate the bake and serve with arugula salad.

Nutrition:

Cal 215

Net Carbs 4g

Fat 15g

Protein 12g

Spanish Paella "Keto-Style"

Preparation time: 10 minutes

Cooking Time: 70 Minutes

Servings: 4

Ingredients:

- 1/2 pound rabbit, cut into pieces
- 1/2 pound chicken drumsticks
- 1 white onion, chopped
- 2 garlic cloves, minced
- 1 red bell pepper, chopped
- 2 tbsp. olive oil 1/2 cup thyme, chopped
- 1 tsp. smoked paprika
- 2 tbsp. tomato puree
- 1/2 cup white wine
- 1 cup chicken broth
- 2 cups cauli rice
- 1 cup green beans, chopped
- A pinch of saffron

Directions:

1. Set oven to 350 F. Warm olive oil in a pan.
2. Fry chicken and rabbit on all sides for 8 minutes; remove to a plate. Attach onion and garlic to the pan and sauté for 3 minutes. Include in tomato puree, bell pepper, and smoked paprika and let

41

simmer for 2 minutes. Pour in broth and simmer for 6 minutes. Stir in cauli rice, white wine, green beans, saffron, and thyme and lay the meat on top.

3. Transfer the pan to the oven and Cooking for 20 minutes. Season and serve.

Nutrition:

Cal 378

Net Carbs 7.6g

Fat 21g

Protein 37g

Basic Chaffles

Preparation Time: 5 minutes

Cooking Time: 6 minutes

Servings: 2

Ingredients:

- 1 large organic egg, beaten
- 1/2 cup Mozzarella cheese, shredded finely

Directions:

1. Preheat a mini Chaffle iron and then grease it.
2. In a small bowl, place the egg and Mozzarella cheese and stir to combine.
3. Set half of the mixture into preheated Chaffle iron and Cooking for about 2-3 minutes or until golden brown.
4. Repeat with the remaining mixture.
5. Serve warm.

Nutrition:

Calories: 56

Net Carb: 0.4g

Fat: 3.7g

Carbohydrates: 0.4g

Dietary Fiber: 0g

Sugar: 0.2g

Protein: 5.2g

Mozzarella Almond Flour Chaffles

Preparation Time: 5 minutes

Cooking Time: 8 minutes

Servings: 2

Ingredients:

- 1/2 cup Mozzarella cheese, shredded
- 1 large organic egg
- 2 tablespoons blanched almond flour
- 1/4 teaspoon organic baking powder

Directions:

1. Preheat a mini Chaffle iron and then grease it.
2. In a medium bowl, attach all ingredients and with a fork, mix until well combined.
3. Set half of the mixture into preheated Chaffle iron and Cooking for about 3-4 minutes.
4. Repeat with the remaining mixture.
5. Serve warm.

Nutrition:

Calories: 98

Net Carb: 1.4g

Fat: 7.1g

Carbohydrates: 2.2g

Dietary Fiber: 0.8g

Sugar: 0.2g

Protein: 6.7g

Simple Cheddar Chaffles

Preparation Time: 5 minutes

Cooking Time: 10 minutes

Servings: 2

Ingredients:

- 1 organic egg, beaten
- 1/2 cup Cheddar cheese, shredded

Directions:

1. Preheat a mini Chaffle iron and then grease it.
2. In a small bowl, add the egg and Mozzarella cheese and stir to combine.
3. Set half of the mixture into preheated Chaffle iron and Cooking for about 3-5 minutes or until golden brown.
4. Repeat with the remaining mixture.
5. Serve warm.

Nutrition:

Calories: 145

Net Carb: 0.5g

Fat: 11.6g

Carbohydrates: 0.5g

Dietary Fiber: 0g

Sugar: 0.3g

Protein: 9.8g

Colby Jack Chaffles

Preparation Time: 5 minutes

Cooking Time: 6 minutes

Servings: 1

Ingredients:

- 2 ounces Colby Jack cheese, sliced thinly in triangles
- 1 large organic egg, beaten

Directions:

1. Preheat a Chaffle iron and then grease it.
2. Arrange 1 thin layer of cheese slices in the bottom of preheated Chaffle iron.
3. Place the beaten egg on top of the cheese.
4. Now, arrange another layer of cheese slices on top to cover evenly.
5. Cooking for about 5-6 minutes.
6. Serve warm.

Nutrition:

Calories: 292

Net Carb: 2.4g

Fat: 23g

Carbohydrates: 9g

Dietary Fiber: 2.4g

Sugar: 0.4g

Protein: 18.3g

Vanilla Colby Jack Chaffles

Preparation Time: 5 minutes

Cooking Time: 6 minutes

Servings: 2

Ingredients:

- 1 large organic egg, beaten
- 1/2 cup Colby Jack cheese, shredded finely
- 1/8 teaspoon organic vanilla extract

Directions:

1. Preheat a mini Chaffle iron and then grease it.
2. In a small bowl, add the egg and Mozzarella cheese and stir to combine.
3. Set half of the mixture into preheated Chaffle iron and Cooking for about 3 minutes or until golden brown.
4. Repeat with the remaining mixture.
5. Serve warm.

Nutrition:

Calories: 147

Net Carb: 1.2g

Fat: 11.5g

Carbohydrates: 1.2g

Dietary Fiber: 0g

Sugar: 0.2g

Protein: 9.2g

Mayonnaise and Cream Cheese Chaffles

Preparation Time: 10 minutes

Cooking Time: 20 minutes

Servings: 4

Ingredients:

- 4 large organic eggs
- 4 tablespoons mayonnaise
- 1 tablespoon almond flour
- 2 tablespoons cream cheese,

Directions:

1. Preheat a Chaffle iron and then grease it.
2. In a bowl, place the eggs, mayonnaise and almond flour and with a hand mixer, mix until smooth.
3. Place about 1/4 of the mixture into preheated Chaffle iron.
4. Place about 1/4 of the cream cheese cubes on top of the mixture evenly and Cooking for about 4-5 minutes or until golden brown.
5. Repeat with the remaining mixture and cream cheese cubes.
6. Serve warm.

Nutrition:

Calories: 190

Net Carb: 0.6g

Fat: 17.7g

Carbohydrates: 0.8g

Dietary Fiber: 0.2g

Sugar: 0.5g

Protein: 6.7g

Mozzarellas and Psyllium Husk Chaffles

Preparation Time: 10 minutes

Cooking Time: 8 minutes

Servings: 2

Ingredients:

- 1/2 cup Mozzarella cheese, shredded
- 1 large organic egg, beaten
- 2 tablespoons blanched almond flour
- 1/2 teaspoon Psyllium husk powder
- 1/4 teaspoon organic baking powder

Directions:

1. Preheat a mini Chaffle iron and then grease it.
2. In a bowl, set all the ingredients and beat until well merged.
3. Set half of the mixture into preheated Chaffle iron and Cooking for about 3-4 minutes or until golden brown.
4. Repeat with the remaining mixture.
5. Serve warm.

Nutrition:

Calories: 101

Net Carb: 1.6g

Fat: 7.1g

Carbohydrates: 2.9g

Dietary Fiber: 1.3g

Sugar: 0.2g

Protein: 6.7g

Layered Cheddar Chaffles

Preparation Time: 5 minutes

Cooking Time: 10 minutes

Servings: 2

Ingredients:

- 1 organic egg, beaten and divided
- 1/2 cup Cheddar cheese

Directions:

1. Preheat a mini Chaffle iron and then grease it.
2. Place about 1/8 cup of cheese in the bottom of the Chaffle iron and top with half of the beaten egg.
3. Now, place 1/8 cup of cheese on top and Cooking for about 4-5 minutes or until golden brown.
4. Repeat with the remaining cheese and egg.
5. Serve warm.

Nutrition:

Calories: 145g

Net Carb: 0.5g

Fat: 11.6g

Carbohydrates: 0.5g

Dietary Fiber: 0g

Sugar: 0.3g

Protein: 9.8g

Layered Two-Cheese Chaffles

Preparation Time: 5 minutes

Cooking Time: 5 minutes

Serving: 1

Ingredients:

- 1 organic egg, beaten
- 1/3 cup Cheddar cheese, shredded
- 1/2 teaspoon ground flaxseed
- 1/4 teaspoon organic baking powder
- 2 tablespoons Parmesan cheese, shredded

Directions:

1. Preheat a mini Chaffle iron and then grease it.
2. In a bowl, set all the ingredients except Parmesan and beat until well combined.
3. Place half the Parmesan cheese in the bottom of preheated Chaffle iron.
4. Place half of the egg mixture over cheese and top with the remaining Parmesan cheese.
5. Cooking for about 3-5 minutes or until golden brown.
6. Serve warm.

Nutrition:

Calories: 264

Net Carb: 1.7g

Fat: 20g

Carbohydrates: 2.1g

Dietary Fiber: 0.4g

Sugar: 0.6g

Protein: 18.9g

Egg-Free Almond Flour Chaffles

Preparation Time: 15 minutes

Cooking Time: 10 minutes

Servings: 2

Ingredients:

- 2 tablespoons cream cheese, softened
- 1 cup Mozzarella cheese, shredded
- 2 tablespoons almond flour
- 1 teaspoon organic baking powder

Directions:

1. Preheat a mini Chaffle iron and then grease it.
2. In a medium bowl, set all ingredients and with a fork, mix until well merged.
3. Set half of the mixture into preheated Chaffle iron and Cooking for about 4-5 minutes or until golden brown.
4. Repeat with the remaining mixture.
5. Serve warm.

Nutrition:

Calories: 77

Net Carb: 2.4g

Fat: 9.8g

Carbohydrates: 3.2g

Dietary Fiber: 0.8g

Sugar: 0.3g

Protein: 4.8g

Egg-Free Psyllium Husk Chaffles

Preparation Time: 5 minutes

Cooking Time: 4 minutes

Serving: 1

Ingredients:

- 1 ounce Mozzarella cheese, shredded
- 1 tablespoon cream cheese, softened
- 1 tablespoon psyllium husk powder

Directions:

1. Preheat a Chaffle iron and then grease it.
2. In a blender, place all ingredients and pulse until a slightly crumbly mixture forms.
3. Place the mixture into preheated Chaffle iron and Cooking for about 3-4 minutes or until golden brown.
4. Serve warm.

Nutrition:

Calories: 137

Net Carb: 1.3g

Fat: 8.8g

Carbohydrates: 1.3g

Dietary Fiber: 0g

Sugar: 0g

Protein: 9.5g

Layered Cheese Chaffles

Preparation time: 8 minutes

Cooking Time: 5 Minutes

Servings: 2

Ingredients:

- 1 organic egg, beaten
- 1/3 cup Cheddar cheese, shredded
- 1/2 teaspoon ground flaxseed
- 1/4 teaspoon organic baking powder
- 2 tablespoons Parmesan cheese, shredded

Directions:

1. Preheat a mini Chaffle iron and then grease it.
2. In a bowl, et all the ingredients except Parmesan and beat until well combined.
3. Place half the Parmesan cheese in the bottom of preheated Chaffle iron.
4. Place half of the egg mixture over cheese and top with the remaining Parmesan cheese.
5. Cooking for about 3-minutes or until golden brown.
6. Serve warm.

Nutrition:

Calories: 264

Net Carb: 1.

Fat: 20g

Saturated Fat: 11.1g

Carbohydrates: 2

Chaffles with Keto Ice Cream

Preparation time: 10 minutes

Cooking Time: 14 Minutes

Servings: 2

Ingredients:

- 1 egg, beaten
- 1/2 cup finely grated mozzarella cheese
- 1/4 cup almond flour
- 2 tbsp. swerve confectioner's sugar
- 1/8 tsp. xanthan gum
- Low-carb ice cream (flavor of your choice) for serving

Directions:

1. Preheat the Chaffle iron.
2. In a medium bowl, merge all the ingredients except the ice cream.
3. Open the iron and add half of the mixture. Close and Cooking until crispy, 7 minutes.
4. Transfer the chaffle to a plate and make second one with the remaining batter.
5. On each chaffle, add a scoop of low carb ice cream, fold into half-moons and enjoy.

Nutrition:

Calories 89

Fats 48g

Carbs 1.67g

Net Carbs 1.37g

Protein 5.91g

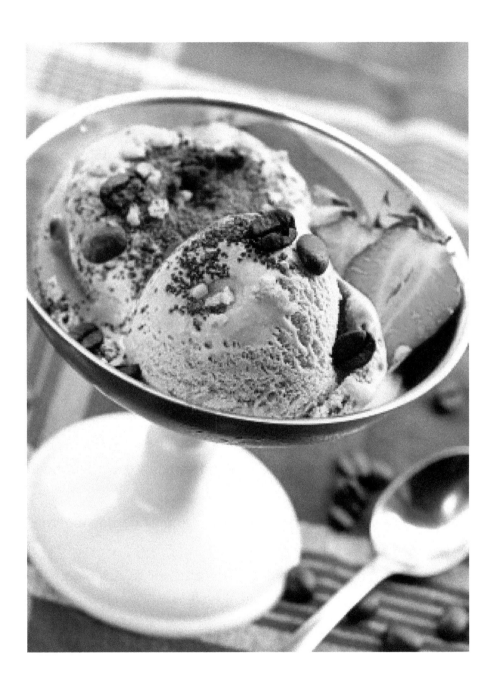

Vanilla Mozzarella Chaffles

Preparation time: 10 minutes

Cooking Time: 12 Minutes

Servings: 2

Ingredients:

- 1 organic egg, beaten
- 1 teaspoon organic vanilla extract
- 1 tablespoon almond flour
- 1 teaspoon organic baking powder
- Pinch of ground cinnamon
- 1 cup Mozzarella cheese, shredded

Directions:

1. Preheat a mini Chaffle iron and then grease it.
2. In a bowl, place the egg and vanilla extract and beat until well combined.
3. Add the flour, baking powder and cinnamon and mix well.
4. Add the Mozzarella cheese and stir to combine.
5. In a small bowl, place the egg and Mozzarella cheese and stir to combine.
6. Set half of the mixture into preheated Chaffle iron and Cooking for about 5-minutes or until golden brown.
7. Repeat with the remaining mixture.

8. Serve warm.

Nutrition:

Calories: 103

Net Carb: 2.4g

Fat: 6.6g

Saturated Fat: 2.3g

Carbohydrates: 2.

Mozzarella and Almond Flour Chaffles

Preparation time: 10 minutes

Cooking Time: 8 Minutes

Servings: 4

Ingredients:

- 1/2 cup Mozzarella cheese, shredded
- 1 large organic egg
- 2 tablespoons blanched almond flour
- 1/4 teaspoon organic baking powder

Directions:

1. Preheat a mini Chaffle iron and then grease it.
2. In a medium bowl, set all ingredients and with a fork, mix until well combined.
3. Set half of the mixture into preheated Chaffle iron and Cooking for about 4 minutes or until golden brown.
4. Repeat with the remaining mixture.
5. Serve warm.

Nutrition:

Calories: 98

Net Carb: 1.4g

Fat: 7.1g

Saturated Fat: 1g

Carbohydrates: 2.2g

Protein: 7g

Cheddar and Egg White Chaffles

Preparation time: 9 minutes

Cooking Time: 12 Minutes

Servings: 2

Ingredients:

- 2 egg whites
- 1 cup Cheddar cheese, shredded

Directions:

1. Preheat a mini Chaffle iron and then grease it.
2. In a small bowl, set the egg whites and cheese and stir to combine.
3. Place 1/4 of the mixture into preheated Chaffle iron and Cooking for about 4 minutes or until golden brown.
4. Repeat with the remaining mixture.
5. Serve warm.

Nutrition:

Calories: 122

Net Carb: 0.5g

Fat: 9.4g

Saturated Fat:

Carbohydrates: 0.5g

Sugar: 0.3g

Protein: 8.8g

Spicy Shrimp and Chaffles

Preparation time: 9 minutes

Cooking Time: 31 Minutes

Servings: 4

Ingredients:

For the shrimp:

- 1 tbsp. olive oil
- 1 lb. jumbo shrimp, peeled and deveined
- 1 tbsp. Creole seasoning
- Salt to taste
- 2 tbsp. hot sauce
- 3 tbsp. butter
- 2 tbsp. chopped fresh scallions to garnish

For the chaffles:

- 2 eggs, beaten
- 1 cup finely grated Monterey Jack cheese

Directions:

For the shrimp:

1. Set the olive oil in a medium skillet over medium heat.
2. Season the shrimp with the Creole seasoning and salt. Cooking in the oil until pink and opaque on both sides, 2 minutes.

3. Pour in the hot sauce and butter. Mix well until the shrimp is adequately coated in the sauce, 1 minute.
4. Turn the heat off and set aside.

For the chaffles:

1. Preheat the Chaffle iron.
2. In a medium bowl, merge the eggs and Monterey Jack cheese.
3. Open the iron and add a quarter of the mixture. Close and Cooking until crispy, 7 minutes.
4. Transfer the chaffle to a plate and make 3 more chaffles in the same manner.
5. Cut the chaffles into quarters and place on a plate.
6. Set with the shrimp and garnish with the scallions.
7. Serve warm.

Nutrition:

Calories 342

Fats 19.75g

Carbs 2.8g

Net Carbs 2.3g

Protein 36.01g

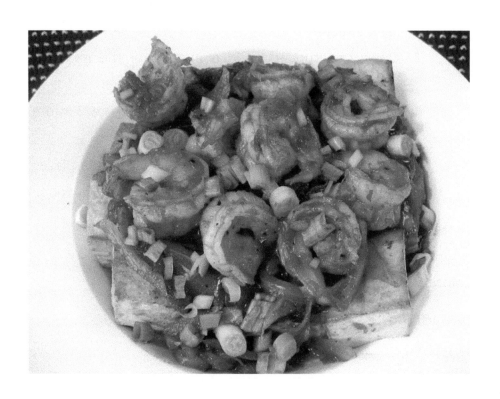

Creamy Chicken Chaffle Sandwich

Preparation time: 10 minutes

Cooking Time: 10 Minutes

Servings: 2

Ingredients:

- Cooking spray
- 1 cup chicken breast fillet, cubed
- Salt and pepper to taste
- 1/4 cup all-purpose cream
- 4 garlic chaffles
- Parsley, chopped

Directions:

1. Spray your pan with oil.
2. Put it over medium heat.
3. Add the chicken fillet cubes.
4. Season with salt and pepper.
5. Reduce heat and add the cream.
6. Spread chicken mixture on top of the chaffle.
7. Garnish with parsley and top with another chaffle.

Nutrition:

Calories 273

Total Fat 34g

Saturated Fat 4.1g

Cholesterol 62mg

Sodium 373mg

Total Carbohydrate 22.5g

Protein 17.5g

Potassium 177mg

Chaffle Cannoli

Preparation time: 9 minutes

Cooking Time: 28 Minutes

Servings: 2

Ingredients:

For the chaffles:

- 1 large egg
- 1 egg yolk
- 3 tbsp. butter, melted
- 1 tbsp. swerve confectioner's
- 1 cup finely grated Parmesan cheese
- 2 tbsp. finely grated mozzarella cheese

For the cannoli filling:

- 1/2 cup ricotta cheese
- 2 tbsp. swerve confectioner's sugar
- 1 tsp. vanilla extract
- 2 tbsp. unsweetened chocolate chips for garnishing

Directions:

1. Preheat the Chaffle iron.
2. Meanwhile, in a medium bowl, merge all the ingredients for the chaffles.
3. Open the iron; pour in a quarter of the mixture, cover, and Cooking until crispy, 7 minutes.

4. Remove the chaffle onto a plate and make 3 more with the remaining batter.
5. Meanwhile, for the cannoli filling:
6. Beat the ricotta cheese and swerve confectioner's sugar until smooth. Mix in the vanilla.
7. On each chaffle, spread some of the filling and wrap over.
8. Garnish the creamy ends with some chocolate chips.
9. Serve immediately.

Nutrition:

Calories 308

Fats 25.05g

Carbs 5.17g

Net Carbs 5.17g

Protein 15.18g

Strawberry Shortcake Chaffle Bowls

Preparation time: 15 minutes

Cooking Time: 28 Minutes

Servings: 2

Ingredients:

- 1 egg, beaten
- 1/2 cup finely grated mozzarella cheese
- 1 tbsp. almond flour
- 1/4 tsp. baking powder
- 2 drops cake batter extract
- 1 cup cream cheese, softened
- 1 cup fresh strawberries, sliced
- 1 tbsp. sugar-free maple syrup

Directions:

1. Preheat a Chaffle bowl maker and grease lightly with Cooking spray.
2. Meanwhile, in a medium bowl, whisk all the ingredients except the cream cheese and strawberries.
3. Open the iron; pour in half of the mixture, cover, and Cooking until crispy, 6 to 7 minutes.
4. Remove the chaffle bowl onto a plate and set aside.
5. Make a second chaffle bowl with the remaining batter.

6. To serve, divide the cream cheese into the chaffle bowls and top with the strawberries.

7. Drizzle the filling with the maple syrup and serve.

Nutrition:

Calories 235

Fats 20.62g

Carbs 5.9g

Net Carbs 5g

Protein 7.51g

Chocolate Melt Chaffles

Preparation time: 9 minutes

Cooking Time: 36 Minutes

Servings: 2

Ingredients:

For the chaffles:

- 2 eggs, beaten
- 1/4 cup finely grated Gruyere cheese
- 2 tbsp. heavy cream
- 1 tbsp. coconut flour
- 2 tbsp. cream cheese, softened
- 3 tbsp. unsweetened cocoa powder
- 2 tsp. vanilla extract
- A pinch of salt

For the chocolate sauce:

- 1/3 cup + 1 tbsp. heavy cream
- 1 1/2 oz. unsweetened baking chocolate, chopped
- 1 1/2 tsp. sugar-free maple syrup
- 1 1/2 tsp. vanilla extract

Directions:

For the chaffles:

1. Preheat the Chaffle iron.

2. In a medium bowl, merge all the ingredients for the chaffles.
3. Open the iron and add a quarter of the mixture. Close and Cooking until crispy, 7 minutes.
4. Transfer the chaffle to a plate and make 3 more with the remaining batter.

For the chocolate sauce:

1. Pour the heavy cream into saucepan and simmer over low heat, 3 minutes.
2. Turn the heat off and attach the chocolate. Allow melting for a few minutes and stir until fully melted, 5 minutes.
3. Mix in the maple syrup and vanilla extract.
4. Assemble the chaffles in layers with the chocolate sauce sandwiched between each layer.
5. Slice and serve immediately.

Nutrition:

Calories 172

Fats 13.57g

Carbs 6.65g

Net Carbs 3.65g

Protein 5.76g

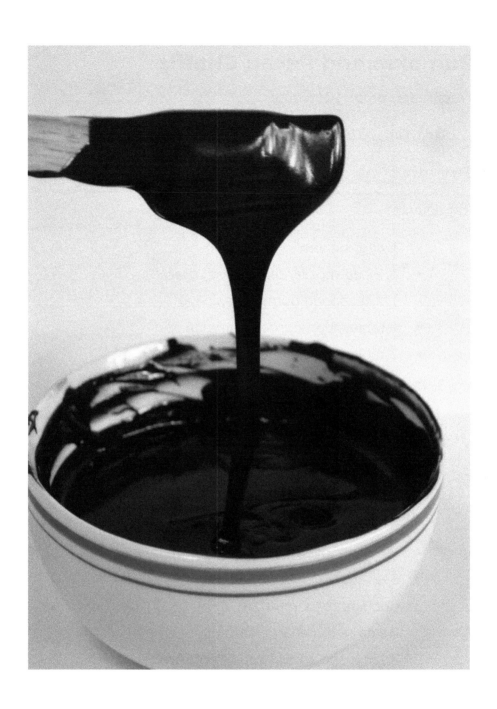

Pumpkin and Pecan Chaffle

Preparation time: 10 minutes

Cooking Time: 10 Minutes

Servings: 2

Ingredients:

- 1 egg, beaten
- 1/2 cup mozzarella cheese, grated
- 1/2 teaspoon pumpkin spice
- 1 tablespoon pureed pumpkin
- 2 tablespoons almond flour
- 1 teaspoon sweetener
- 2 tablespoons pecans, chopped

Directions:

1. Turn on the Chaffle maker.
2. Beat the egg in a bowl.
3. Stir in the rest of the ingredients.
4. Pour half of the mixture into the device.
5. Seal the lid.
6. Cooking for 5 minutes.
7. Remove the chaffle carefully.
8. Repeat the steps to make the second chaffle.

Nutrition:

Calories 210

Total Fat 17 g

Saturated Fat 10 g

Cholesterol 110 mg

Sodium 250 mg

Potassium 570 mg

Total Carbohydrate 4.6 g

Spicy Jalapeno and Bacon Chaffles

Preparation time: 10 minutes

Servings: 2

Cooking Time: 5 Minutes

Ingredients:

- 1 oz. cream cheese
- 1 large egg
- 1/2 cup cheddar cheese
- 2 tbsps. bacon bits
- 1/2 tbsp. jalapenos
- 1/4 tsp. baking powder

Directions:

1. Switch on your Chaffle maker.
2. Set your Chaffle maker with Cooking spray and let it heat up.
3. Mix together egg and vanilla extract in a bowl first.
4. Add baking powder, jalapenos and bacon bites.
5. Add in cheese last and mix together.
6. Pour the chaffles batter into the maker and Cooking the chaffles for about 2-3 minutes
7. Once chaffles are Coo kinged, remove from the maker.
8. Serve hot and enjoy!

Nutrition:

Protein: 24

Fat: 70

Carbohydrates: 6

Zucchini Parmesan Chaffles

Preparation time: 10 minutes

Cooking Time: 14 Minutes

Servings: 2

Ingredients:

- 1 cup shredded zucchini
- 1 egg, beaten
- 1/2 cup finely grated Parmesan cheese
- Salt and freshly ground black pepper

Directions:

1. Preheat the Chaffle iron.
2. Set all the ingredients in a bowl and mix well.
3. Open the iron and add half of the mixture. Close and Cooking until crispy, 7 minutes.
4. Remove the chaffle onto a plate and make another with the remaining mixture.
5. Cut each chaffle into wedges and serve afterward.

Nutrition:

Calories 138

Fats 9.07g

Carbs 3.81g

Net Carbs 3.71g

Protein 10.02g

Cheddar and Almond Flour Chaffles

Preparation time: 10 minutes

Cooking Time: 10 Minutes

Servings: 2

Ingredients:

- 1 large organic egg, beaten
- 1/2 cup Cheddar cheese, shredded
- 2 tablespoons almond flour

Directions:

1. Preheat a mini Chaffle iron and then grease it.
2. In a bowl, place the egg, Cheddar cheese and almond flour and beat until well merged.
3. Set half of the mixture into preheated Chaffle iron and Cooking for about 5 minutes or until golden brown.
4. Repeat with the remaining mixture.
5. Serve warm.

Nutrition:

Calories: 195

Net Carb: 1g

Fat: 15.Saturated

Fat: 7g

Carbohydrates: 1.8g

Dietary Fiber: 0.8g

Sugar: 0.6g

Protein: 10.2g

Simple and Beginner Chaffle

Preparation time: 10 minutes

Servings: 2

Cooking Time: 5 Minutes

Ingredients:

- 1 large egg
- 1/2 cup mozzarella cheese, shredded
- Cooking spray

Directions:

1. Switch on your Chaffle maker.
2. Set the egg with a fork in a small mixing bowl.
3. Once the egg is beaten, add the mozzarella and mix well.
4. Spray the Chaffle maker with Cooking spray.
5. Pour the chaffles mixture in a preheated Chaffle maker and let it Cooking for about 2-3 minutes.
6. Once the chaffles are cooked, carefully remove them from the maker and Cooking the remaining batter.
7. Serve hot with coffee and enjoy!

Nutrition:

Protein: 36

Fat: 60

Carbohydrates: 4

Asian Cauliflower Chaffles

Preparation time: 9 minutes

Cooking Time: 28 Minutes

Servings: 2

Ingredients:

For the chaffles:

- 1 cup cauliflower rice, steamed
- 1 large egg
- Salt and freshly ground black pepper
- 1 cup finely grated Parmesan cheese
- 1 tsp. sesame seeds
- 1/4 cup chopped fresh scallions

For the dipping sauce:

- 3 tbsp. coconut aminos
- 1 1/2 tbsp. plain vinegar
- 1 tsp. fresh ginger puree
- 1 tsp. fresh garlic paste
- 3 tbsp. sesame oil
- 1 tsp. fish sauce
- 1 tsp. red chili flakes

Directions:

1. Preheat the Chaffle iron.

2. In a medium bowl, mix the cauliflower rice, egg, salt, black pepper, and Parmesan cheese.
3. Open the iron and add a quarter of the mixture. Close and Cooking until crispy, 7 minutes.
4. Transfer the chaffle to a plate and make 3 more chaffles in the same manner.
5. Meanwhile, make the dipping sauce.
6. In a medium bowl, merge all the ingredients for the dipping sauce.
7. Plate the chaffles, garnish with the sesame seeds and scallions and serve with the dipping sauce.

Nutrition:

Calories 231

Fats 188g

Carbs 6.32g

Net Carbs 5.42g

Protein 9.66g

Sharp Cheddar Chaffles

Preparation time: 10 minutes

Cooking Time: 10 Minutes

Servings: 2

Ingredients:

- 1 organic egg, beaten
- 1/2 cup sharp Cheddar cheese, shredded

Directions:

1. Preheat a mini Chaffle iron and then grease it.
2. In a small bowl, place the egg and cheese and stir to combine.
3. Set half of the mixture into preheated Chaffle iron and Cooking for about 5 minutes or until golden brown.
4. Repeat with the remaining mixture.
5. Serve warm.

Nutrition:

Calories: 145

Net Carb: 0.5g

Fat: 11.Saturated

Fat: 6.6g

Carbohydrates: 0.5g

Sugar: 0.3g

Protein: 9.8g

Keto-Bread Twists

Preparation Time: 20 minutes

Cooking Time: 20 minutes

Servings: 6

Ingredients

- 1/4 cup almond flour
- 2 Tbsp. coconut flour
- 1/2 tsp. salt
- 1/2 Tbsp. baking powder
- 1/2 cup cheese, shredded
- 2 Tbsp. butter
- 2 eggs
- 1/4 cup green pesto

Directions

1. Preheat the oven to 350F and prepare a baking tray.
2. Combine coconut flour, almond flour, baking powder, and salt in a bowl.
3. Mix butter, cheese, and egg in another bowl.
4. Combine the flour mixture with the butter mixture and form dough.
5. Take 2 parchment sheets and place the dough in between them.
6. Set the dough into a rectangular shape with a rolling pin and remove the parchment paper from one side.

7. Drizzle the green pesto on the loaf and cut it into strips and twist them.
8. Put the baking tray in the oven and bake for 20 minutes.
9. Remove from oven and serve.

Nutrition:

Calories: 151

Fat: 12.9g

Carb: 3.5g

Protein: 5.8g

Bruleed French Toast Chaffle Monte Cristo

Preparation time: 10 minutes

Cooking time: 5 minutes

Servings: 1

Ingredients:

- 1 egg
- 1/8 tsp. baking powder
- 1/4 tsp. cinnamon
- 1/2 tsp. monk fruit
- 1 tbsp. cream cheese
- 2 tsp. brown sugar substitute
- 2 oz. deli ham
- 2 oz. deli turkey
- 1 slice provolone cheese
- 1/2 tsp. sugar-free jelly

Directions:

1. Preheat the Chaffle maker.
2. Place all the chaffle ingredients, except the sugar substitute, inside a blender. Make sure to place the cream cheese closest to the blades. Blend the ingredients until you achieve a smooth consistency.

3. Sprinkle the Chaffle maker with 1/2 tsp. of brown sugar substitute.

4. Onto the Chaffle maker, pour 1/2 of the batter. Sprinkle another 1/2 teaspoon of the brown sugar substitute.

5. Secure the lid and allow the batter to Cooking for 3-5 minutes.

6. Remove the chaffle. Repeat the steps until you used up all the batter.

7. Prepare the chaffle by spreading jelly on one surface of the chaffle.

8. Following this order, place the ham, turkey, and cheese in a small, microwaveable bowl. Place inside the microwave. Heat until the cheese is melted.

9. Invert the bowl onto the chaffle so that the contents transfer onto the chaffle. The cheese should be under the ham and turkey, directly sitting on top of the chaffle.

10. Top with the other chaffle and flip it over before serving.

Nutrition:

Calories: 368

Carbohydrate: 7g

Fat: 22g

Protein: 34g

Avocado and Mushroom Pizza Cups

Preparation time: 9 minutes

Cooking Time: 35 Minutes

Servings: 4

Ingredients:

- 1/2 cup sliced mushrooms
- 1 1/2 cups cauli rice
- 1 tbsp. olive oil
- 2 cups pizza sauce
- 1 cup grated Monterey Jack
- 1 cup grated mozzarella
- 2 large tomatoes, chopped
- 1 small red onion, chopped
- 1 tsp. dried oregano
- 2 jalapeño peppers, chopped
- 1 avocado, chopped
- 2 tbsp. water
- 1/4 cup chopped cilantro
- Salt and black pepper to taste

Directions:

1. Preheat oven to 400 F. Microwave cauli rice for 2 minutes. Fluff with a fork and set aside. Brush 4 ramekins with olive oil and spread half of the pizza

sauce at the bottom. Top with half of cauli rice and half of the cheeses.

2. In a bowl, mix mushrooms, tomatoes, onion, oregano, jalapeños, salt, and pepper. Scoop half of the mixture into the ramekins and repeat the layering process, finishing off with cheese. Bake for 20 minutes.

3. Top with avocado and cilantro.

Nutrition:

Cal 378

Net Carbs 3.4g

Fat 22g

Protein 21g

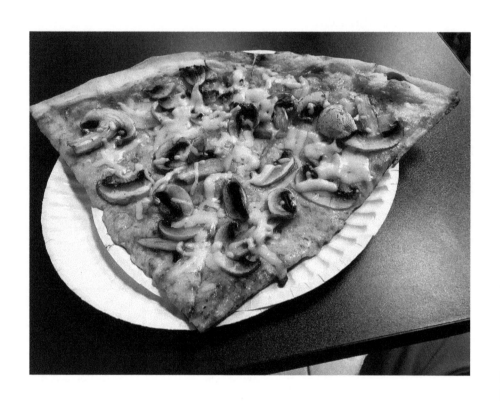

Broccoli Slaw with Pecans

Preparation time: 9 minutes

Cooking Time: 28 Minutes

Servings: 4

Ingredients:

- 2 tbsp. olive oil
- 2 cups broccoli slaw
- 1 red bell pepper, sliced
- 1 red onion, thinly sliced
- 1/2 cup toasted pecans, chopped
- 2 tbsp. flax seeds
- 1 tbsp. red wine vinegar
- 1/2 lemon, juiced
- 1 tsp. Dijon mustard
- 2 tbsp. mayonnaise
- 2 tbsp. chopped cilantro
- Salt and black pepper to taste

Directions:

1. In a bowl, thoroughly combine broccoli slaw, bell pepper, red onion, cilantro, salt, and pepper. Mix in pecans and flax seeds. In another small bowl, whisk the red wine vinegar, olive oil, lemon juice, mayonnaise, and mustard.
2. Drizzle the dressing over the slaw and serve.

Nutrition:

Cal 198

Net Carbs 1.6g

Fat 15g

Protein 10

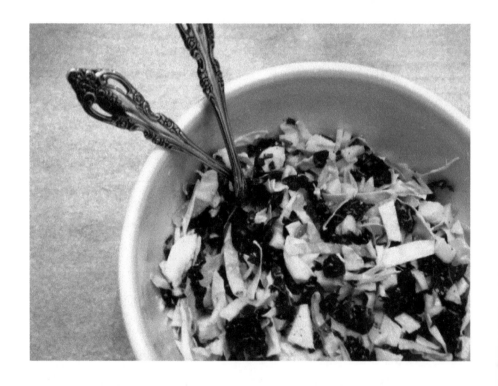